My Journey to Better Health

My Personal Journey to Wellness and Understanding My Body

Shawna Boudreaux

ISBN: 978-1-7361117-6-5 (Paperback)

ISBN: 978-1-7361117-7-2 (Digital)

All rights reserved. No part of this publication may be reproduced, or transmitted in any form or by any means, including photocopying, recording, or other electronic or mechanical methods without the prior written permission of the publisher. For permission requests, solicit the publisher via the email address below.

SG Boudreaux

P.O. Box 12936

Lake Charles, La. 70612

Printed in the USA

Sgboodro2@yahoo.com

www.SGBoudreaux.com

Copyright © year 2022 by SG Boudreaux

All rights reserved

Shawna Boudreaux

Table of Contents

Chapter	Page
1 My Story Begins	1
2 The Next Twenty Years	23
3 Faith's Story	37
4 People	57
5 Levels of Health	63
6 Trying New Things	69
7 Paying Attention	75
8 Being Content	79
About the Author	84

Introduction

Hello, my name is Shawna Boudreaux. I first started writing clean, faith-based, fiction, and fantasy novels back in 2017 under the pen name S.G. Boudreaux. However, after much nudging from the Lord, the book you are about to read is an explanation of my health journey from an early age to present day, and my still constantly changing health. What I have discovered over the last forty years or so has led me down many pathways and has brought me to my current state of being; right where God has placed me. I am much better than I was, but still struggle at times to figure out my ever-changing body. But without the Lord's leading I would not be where I am today. I am reminded of what *Romans 8:28 says:*

> *And we know that in all things that God works for the good for those who love Him, who have been called according to His purpose.*

Does this mean my fiction writing days are over? Of course not; even now I am writing another story as I switch between the facts of life and the escape to fantasy. Fiction, fantasy, and adventure are too much fun to write to just stop, and I truly feel that God led me to write in those genres to offer clean-reading and God honoring options for others as well, and as a Christian, I can't write contrary to my beliefs. But, God has impressed upon me the need to tell my story in the hopes that it may help someone else find their healing journey. Has my journey been life threatening? No, not really, and it doesn't deal with anything like cancer, thank the Lord, although I came very close to that possibility at one point just a few years back; again God spared me this. But I have had my share of illness and debilitating disease that has prevented me from living an active, full life like I have wanted. It has affected career choices, hobbies, travels, friendships, and even the lives of those in my immediate family. I hope that reading about my story will somehow help you with your own and give you some knowledge about how to start or continue your own healing journey. At the very least, you will find a sympathetic heart to affirm that you're not alone in the craziness of health issues.

Inside, you will also find a contribution chapter by one of my sisters whom I mention in the book, Faith. I asked her to provide her own story and journey as well, and I hope you can glean inspiration or help from the information we have provided.

Blessings,

Shawna

My Journey to Better Health

Chapter 1

My Story Begins

Before I start, I will say that the first three chapters will be considerably longer than the rest, as I and my sister set the stage of our own personal stories and journeys with our health.

I was like most healthy kids, always running and doing things, mostly all day, every day. Growing up in the hollers and mountains of West Virginia we had a certain level of freedom, but that is another story; one which I hope to write one day with my many sisters and only brother.

My health problems started around late middle school when I was about thirteen-years-old, where I began to have many different health issues. There is only a small time in my past that I haven't dealt with some form of ailment; between my birth and becoming a teenager.

I started my menstrual cycle at the age of eleven, and they were normal for many years. As I got into high school I started having horrible pain and heavy bleeding. Then, as I got a bit older I started having gut issues on top of that; problems with extreme constipation. Because of this constipation, I would get nausea, pain, and just feel sick. Doctors ran a few minor tests but found nothing wrong with me. My

My Journey to Better Health

problems weren't severe or frequent enough to make me terribly ill, but enough for such discomfort that the intense pain in my lower left side around the top of my hip bone would immobilize me at times. Often times this would happen while at school, I would get to first- or second-hour classes and have to leave because I was in so much pain that it would make me throw up.

I wasn't an unhealthy girl. I ate well and got plenty of exercise, but I did have an unusual amount of stress in my life; more so than your average teenager, but that too is another story. At first I attributed my problems to this stress, but later realized that was not the case.

As time went by, my gut problems only escalated; to add to that, I began to have severe menstrual cycles. At times they were very heavy and lasted several weeks, and at other times they were normal and lasted only days.

As a senior in high school, looking to find my way and my future, I had at one point decided to become a helicopter pilot for the US Airforce. I was excited about this, but soon realized that I could not seek such a profession. My stomach issues were too severe, and at the moment uncontrollable. I would have never made it through basic training, and so I had to change my direction.

When my health issues began to escalate in severity, people, often adults, accused me of lying because they couldn't see anything wrong with me. Even physicians thought I was making things up just so I didn't have to attend school. I liked school. It was an escape for me; again, another story. Some people might have even called me a hypochondriac, but all of my health issues have been very real. There have been varying stages of the same problems. My gut issues would stop for a few months or so, only to return later. This did not help exonerate me with the people that thought I was lying or exaggerating my sickness. Some of my health issues have gone away, mainly because the offending body part has been removed. That in itself has caused its own issues. I will elaborate more on how this affected me later in the book.

When I became an adult at around eighteen-years-of-age, my menstrual cycle became worse, and my gut issues worsened as well, causing me to have to take medications to help with the symptoms. This started an avalanche of prescriptions from the big drug companies. I have even tried bio-identical medicines made specifically for my chemical make-up from our local homeopathic drugstores. I have tried several different avenues in an attempt to find a solution to satisfy my body's issues. I have had some very odd reactions to most of these medications, both manmade and natural. My siblings, like myself, generally have adverse reactions to the typical fixes in medicine as well. The things that generally help most everyone else can cause problems for us. I'll speak more on this as well as the story progresses.

I mentioned earlier that I grew up in West Virginia, but when my father died when I was nine, my mother could not make a living there, and so we moved to Florida three years later when I was twelve, and we lived there until I was eighteen. It was at that age when life's struggles moved us again. We left Florida and moved to Lake Charles, Louisiana. At that point, Mom was a single mother with one

My Journey to Better Health

younger child still left to raise, living on my father's social security check and what little she could earn from working. I often pitched in wherever I could to help pay bills and tend to the needs of my youngest sister. During this time my health became much worse. There were days that I couldn't even get out of bed the pain in my stomach was so bad. Those days usually coincided with my menstrual cycle. I had some normal cycles that weren't so bad and lasted about a week or so, even though I still had heavy bleeding and clotting. But on the days that moving was difficult and very painful, my cycles were extremely heavy and would often last for three weeks. This frequently caused stabbing pains in my lower abdomen, as well as lower back pain and achy legs; sometimes it would cause me to run a fever. If not working, I would often lay in bed or on the couch for hours with a heating pad several days in a row. I lived on Advil, the normal medications for heavy menstrual cycles did not help me at all. On top of that, my stomach issues worsened with a horrible pain in my left side that stopped me in my tracks, bending me over trying to catch my breath, and causing me to throw up. It seemed like my body was fighting against itself. Each issue vying for the opportunity to prove it had the upper hand and could do the most damage.

We had no medical insurance and lived on a very tight budget. Fortunately, Lake Charles offered a charity hospital that I was able to take advantage of in an attempt to figure out what was happening to me; unfortunately with very little success. Charity—as much of a blessing as it was—was also many hours of waiting. I would spend countless nights in the waiting room of the charity hospital, often getting out of bed in the middle of the night because the pain was so bad I couldn't sleep. Fortunately, I had my own car and could drive myself as Mom had work the next morning and my youngest sister had school. I would wake Mom to tell her where I was going or leave her a note so she wouldn't worry.

The waiting room of the charity hospital was on these nights barren of people. Only a handful of us sat waiting to be seen, some passed out in a chair. Even with as few as that, the waiting still took many hours. Other times, during regular daylight hours, the waiting room was littered with people, some had to stand as seating was full while others lay on the outdoor lawn, or sat in other shady areas around the building, all within earshot of the waiting rooms intercom system. During this time when the place was packed, the waiting felt endless as it took hours—and sometimes days—to see the financial department to see if I would even qualify for assistance, and then hours more to see an actual doctor. Once I finally was able to see a doctor, I then had to be referred to another physician in a field of medical expertise needed for my issue. These appointments were often spaced months apart, but again, the care and treatment was free. I learned to deal with my illness because I had no other choice but to wait. Eventually I sought out professionals myself and paid out of pocket for these visits because, again, the doctors at the charity facility couldn't find anything wrong with me.

Based on my symptoms, I was referred to a specialist; a gastroenterologist; and I was eventually diagnosed with IBS—Irritable Bowel Syndrome—simply through speaking with the doctor. I was prescribed medicine to help with

My Journey to Better Health

my gut issues of pain, constipation, and throwing up. Some of these medications worked for a few months, and others only worked a few days. I went through several prescriptions over a year or so, trying to find something that would work long enough to get some relief, but my body would develop a tolerance to whatever I was taking and the medicine would stop working all together.

At this time I was also going to a gynecologist for my painful female issues. There were times when it felt as though a knife had been plunged into my lower abdomen or vaginal area. After an internal ultrasound which led to exploratory surgery, my gynecologist stated that my left ovary was stuck to the back of my uterus, but it appeared to be working fine so there was no need for surgery. I thought at the time that his diagnosis of "it was fine" sounded strange, but I was no doctor, so I didn't question it. To control the problems with the heavy bleeding and often extremely painful cycles, I was given birth control pills to lessen the effects of my menstrual cycle issues. Fortunately, they did the job nicely as far as my female issues went and life was normal, for a time. Little did I know that these birth control pills would cause my IBS issues to worsen.

One particular day, not to long after moving to Louisiana, I remember being so sick, feeling as though I was running a fever so Mom took me to town to see a doctor. I don't remember the diagnosis, probably something like a virus because nothing else was done for me. This trip was made worse because Mom's little car was on its last leg, and she needed a new one. While she wheeled and dealed with a salesman at a local car lot for a newer, more dependable, and affordable vehicle, I laid in the back of Mom's dilapidated car in the middle of the Louisiana summer heat, horribly ill. Even though I was sick, she needed a new car. Mine was a manual shift and she had never learned to drive one. I don't think her current vehicle would have even gotten us home that day. I remember us having trouble getting it started at the charity hospital, needing help to do so, spurring her to stop at the car lot. She did manage to get a better vehicle and I survived the torturous afternoon. I think the salesman felt sorry for her being a single mother, and with me lying ill in the back seat, cut her a pretty sweet deal.

This having been just another example of Romans 8:28 and God's loving hand in my life.

As a young adult these symptoms and ailments made work hard for me. But through the grace of God I managed it and I worked a lot. I waited tables on split shifts five days a week, a long day on the sixth and off one day. "Splits", as they were called, consisted of the hours from nine a.m. to two p.m., then again from four p.m. to eleven p.m.; often an hour or so later for cleanup. I managed it well when I was young. When my stomach would act up, often at work because that is where I usually was, it would incapacitate me. I was frozen in place, bent over in such horrid pain that it hurt to breathe, so I would try to hold my breath until a time presented itself that I could move without too much pain. I would then have to find a restroom, throwing up while I sat on the toilet with cramping from constipation until my bowels would decide to move. I tried not to show that I was in pain to anyone. I had always been good at hiding things, mainly because I didn't want to bother others, and frankly, what

My Journey to Better Health

could they do when doctors couldn't help me? Most of my fellow employees were ignorant of my stomach issues, until a time when they saw me bent over for a minute or two and supporting myself as I clung to an obliging counter or wall. These pains, once I threw up and my stomach emptied, would just go away with no other ill effects. I then would just go on with my day as normal, because for me, it was.

At one point this happened so frequently that I had to ask my boss to lay me off. Thank goodness I had a wonderful boss who liked me because, even though I had health issues, I was a good, hard-working, honest, employee. For four months I could not work, and because of the lack of work, I also ended up pawning off just about everything I owned for money. My unemployment was only twenty-dollars a week since I was a waitress and minimum wage for that profession was two dollars and twenty-five cents an hour back then.

Brief off subject tirade for a moment; did you know that waiters and waitresses made so little? The last time I checked they still only make about four dollars and twenty-five cents an hour, so be nice and tip the person waiting on your table.

Sorry, small but important deviation there.

Anyway, on top of work I also attended business school for a year, working two separate waitress positions in the process. I never had a day off, and yet, during that time in my life, I don't recall my symptoms being as bad. Like I said before, there were times when I had very little trouble with my health, and times when it stopped my life almost completely. I can't explain what the difference was; I just know that I was happy for the reprieve when I got one.

As I mentioned earlier, I was also being seen by a gynecologist, not associated with the charity hospital, he was an out-of-pocket visit. But with my symptoms getting worse I went back to the charity hospital in Lake Charles and was referred to the charity hospital in Lafayette. My physician there was shocked by my diagnosis. He said that I had a vaginal mass the size of a softball and that surgical removal was necessary. I asked if they could do a bikini cut on my abdomen to minimize scarring but was told no. The mass was so large it had grown out of the top of my uterus and had wrapped around the outside of my uterine wall. Because they did not know what else they would find upon opening up my uterine area, the incision would have to be from the navel down.

Here's a little fun story for you. Now since this was a learning hospital for the local college students, all patients were fair game. I had been examined by another young doctor in training because the physician who was training him, was so shocked by the size of the mass inside me he wanted the other doctor to see it for himself. Talk about feeling like you're on display. Geesh! But I agreed. Who was I to stand in the way of science? Besides, I was getting free care. Hopefully that young man actually learned something useful. Besides, I was used to being poked and prodded from early on. Humbled, I most certainly was.

After surgery, I was told that the fibroid tumor; non-cancerous; was so large that it had begun to decay in the center, and that it was equivalent in size to my being five-months pregnant. I had a baby fibroid! I also asked

My Journey to Better Health

about the ovary that my gynecologist had said was stuck to the back of my uterus and the doctor said that was not the case. My ovaries were where they were supposed to be. Apparently what my gynecologist had seen was the fibroid mass. Needless to say, I never went back to that gynecologist; I found a new one. This alone was not the only reason I left the man's care; I also had another friend who experienced strange practices with this same doctor which I did not agree with.

The Lafayette surgeon then also told me because of the mass and damage to my body, and the fact that I had some endometriosis, another culprit to all the pain I was having, I would likely never have children. There was a fifty-fifty chance, but he believed and stressed to me that I would likely never be able to get pregnant. Because of the endometriosis that also plagued my insides, they left me on the birth-control pills to help to regulate and minimize my still heavy menstrual cycles.

Well, at least my cycles were now more regular and the occasional stabbing and debilitating pain was now gone. Life was good for a while, until my gut would take more bouts of extreme pain and nausea. I would be fine one minute and doubled over the next; unable to breathe normally or move for several minutes. The pain in my left side was so horrendous I felt like I was in the movie alien and something foreign could come bursting out of me at any moment. No joke, it was that bad. I once explained to my gastroenterologist that it felt as though I was having labor pains, even though I had never experienced childbirth. He said that many people related having the same sort of pain. Believe it or not, again, my gastroenterologist could find nothing wrong with me. Even after a colonoscopy around the age of twenty-three. He reiterated that it was just the symptoms of Irritable Bowel Syndrome and I would just have to live with the pain and take medication to help control it.

Wow! What every young woman wants to hear for the rest of her life, right?

But I am getting ahead of myself here. Let me go back to age nineteen.

After my fibroid removal we moved back to Florida for about a year. We were staying with my eldest sister and her husband until we could find a place to live. While taking an afternoon nap one day, I awoke to a pain so severe in my chest that I literally thought I was having a heart attack at my young age.

Mom rushed me to the local charitable hospital, and they told her it was nerves and stress causing my problem. They gave me a shot and a little while later I was fine. Did I agree with their diagnosis? No I did not and even voiced my opinion to the nurses and doctor. At that point in my life I was the most unstressed I had been since I was eight-years-old. I explained this to them and they just brushed it off. Their efforts did end my pain however and we went home. Not long after that, I had another attack; the pain was the same as before. It hurt badly through my chest and upper-back, lasting for hours, with no relief. I felt as though I couldn't breathe, and nothing eased or stopped the excruciating squeezing pain except whatever medicine the clinic gave me for anxiety.

Later, I went to the walk-in clinic again to have another go at trying to figure out what was wrong with me. The physician on call was a

My Journey to Better Health

foreign doctor and extremely rude to me, basing his opinion solely on my appearance. He looked over my small chart, looked me up and down and rudely told me to go home. He said there was nothing wrong with me, I was healthy and young, and wasting their time. I was dumbfounded and very angry, and expressed my thoughts to a nurse with no recourse. So, I went home and got on with life, until I had another attack. I went back to the same clinic and the attending physician on rotation that day was also training another younger doctor. This attending physician actually paid attention to me, coming to a conclusion and diagnosis as I explained that I had a family history of early onset gallbladder disease or gall stones. He was able to diagnose gallbladder disease after listening to me; telling the trainee that if you only listen to your patients, they will often tell you what is wrong with them. Thank God for placing this man at the clinic on that particular day. He then told me that I had all the symptoms but none of the conditions that would cause the disease, meaning it was likely hereditary. I was young, thin, had never been pregnant; not counting the fibroid of course; and was relatively healthy. But, because my father and two of my older sisters had their gall bladders removed before the age of thirty, I likely had the disease as well.

He had listened to me and what I had to say, taking my history into account. This doctor referred me to another wonderful doctor who treated me until I could get an appointment with a gastroenterologist. It is amazing the results you can get when you find a knowledgeable doctor that cares, will consider that you have an issue, and is willing to pursue it. So, take heart if you are in the same situation. There is a doctor that God will guide you to that will help you to overcome your issues. But first, you must have a personal relationship with God, and be willing to ask and listen. God is not a genie in a bottle at your disposal, beck, and call. He is a caring loving Father who knows better what you need than you do.

I lived with this suddenly occurring, obstructive pain for three to four months on medication and a special diet until my then physician could refer me to a gastroenterologist through yet another charitable medical organization. I was already a tiny person, but during that time I could have no fat in my diet at all since this spurred my gallbladder into action. I lived on baked, skinless, boneless, bland, chicken breast with just a very small pinch of salt to taste, and that was all. I was literally withering away, but I continued on with my life, a little better for the knowledge if a little worse for wear. While I worked and waited to get an appointment with the aforementioned charity organization, so that I could get a permanent resolution to my presumed gallbladder issue, my living with this way of life did help. I didn't have too many attacks that were severe and I even felt well enough to participate in a TV dance show in Tampa, Florida. I know, I was very sick, but I was also young, strong, and determined to live life a fully as I was aloud.

So, while out dancing in a club one night, I was approached by a man who searched the local dance clubs for dancers to participate in his show. My dancing for this TV show only lasted a month or two and I quickly quit that for moral issues. It was an interesting experience,

My Journey to Better Health

but one that when realized can be easily walked away from; a definite learning curve for a Godly young woman raised in church all her life.

Now remember, I still suffered with my IBS issues through all of this as well. That never went away, only eased at times. Mostly, I felt absolutely fine, but that could quickly change, and I couldn't always find a reason for the unexpected flair-up.

To continue; I eventually got my appointment with the charity organization and was referred to a gastroenterologist. This was great news, but I was also reserved after my initial visit with the doctor, because he told me that I had gallbladder disease and would have to have it removed. Now, my father had been a relatively healthy man, but also had had his share of illnesses. He had gone through several surgeries and had a scar that resembled a cross from his chest to his abdomen, and a huge scar that wrapped around his right side from his gallbladder removal. I remembered daddy's chest and right side vividly and I did not want that scar, but what choice did I have? Fortunately for me, the gastroenterologist was starting a new procedure and I was a prime candidate. An outpatient surgery for removal of the gall bladder which required three small incisions made to the skin. Thin tubes were then inserted and the removal was done by way of the tubes. They made one incision for the laser, one for the camera, and one for the removal. The laser burned the organ off and it was suctioned out through the tube. They literally put three little band-aids on my incisions and sent me home that afternoon. Thank goodness for medical advances, saving me from the horrible scarring and the weeks without work. God's timing indeed. I was even given a VHS tape of the surgery to watch later; which I couldn't bring myself to do for a long time. My brother had asked to watch it and thought it was totally amazing, and so eventually convinced me to watch it as well. It was gruesome I tell you, especially since I knew this was done inside of me. It even made me dizzy and a bit nauseous to see. But it also amazes me how these doctors can learn to do what they do for ease and patient benefit. The surgery was a complete success and I was able to eat and live pain free from the evil gall stones, and all with just three little scars no longer than paper cuts.

Unfortunately this did not solve my gut issues. When we left Florida again to return to Louisiana, I was a bit better due to the care I had received in Florida. But I still had horrible stomach issues with intense pain and throwing up, and this would continue for many years in varying stages of severity. It even seemed as though they were worse than ever before. But as my Lake Charles gastroenterologist stated, I would just have to live with it. And I did; through marriage at twenty-five, and through pregnancy at twenty-six. Thank goodness my stomach attacks weren't severe at that time. I had stopped taking birth control when I got married because we wanted to have children, even though I was told I never would. I knew there was always the chance and that if we didn't try, I would never know for sure. I knew my God, and that man cannot speak against Him.

My Journey to Better Health

Matthew 19:26 says:

> *And looking at them, Jesus said to them, "with people this is impossible, but with God all things are possible."*

Even though I wanted children, at the same time I was terrified to have them because of my health issues. I was also concerned about the irregularity and pain of my cycles returning, but only three months after stopping the birth control, I became pregnant. I was excited and fearful at the same time. I was excited because I could have children; the doctor had been wrong, and I was also fearful for my child. What if I had the IBS attacks while pregnant? Would I miscarry the baby? Not only that, but I had these awful fears that I would pass on this horrible debilitating disease to my children. I did not want any future children to have to deal with such unrelenting pain for the rest of their lives too. I was so concerned by this that at one point I thought about not chancing pregnancy and only adopting.

My pregnancy went great by the way, although I did have a weird temporary, and again, unexplainable thing happen with my vision, where I had straight on blind spots and squiggly electrical looking white lines around my vision center. It only lasted a few days, and after being checked by an optician, was told my vision was perfect and they could not explain what had happened. I only experienced this phenomenon one other time in my life, much later on during the solar eclipse of 2017. Only, during the eclipse I also had migraines to go along with the squiggles. This lasted for two weeks prior to the eclipse and I have not experienced it since. I know-weird right? But, we are God's creations, just like the sun, moon, and stars. The moon controls the tides so why would we too not be affected by such things? I read somewhere recently, that since are bodies are made mostly of water, why would the moon not affect us?

Nehemiah 9:6 tells us:

> *You alone are the LORD. You made the heavens even the highest heavens, and all their starry host the earth and all that is on it, the sea and all that is in them You give life to everything, and the multitudes of heaven worship you.*

Think about that verse for a moment. God designed everything to work together. Pay attention to your body during different elemental occurrences, you might just discover a pattern to some of your own issues.

Now, during my pregnancy, I also had a slipped disk in my back from working seventy-hours a week while pregnant in our little local take-out only restaurant. I had worked this way before pregnancy so why not continue. However, I had to stop this and stay home and not work at all. Eventually over the course of a month or two the disk just went back into place all on its own. After my daughter's birth, I had to stop working all together and we had to close down our take-out kitchen for good. There was

My Journey to Better Health

no way I would be able to work like that with a newborn, and my husband had his own full-time job to tend to.

For my delivery, my new OB/GYN would not allow me to deliver naturally, even though I tried to get him to let me, citing all the articles I had read in pregnancy magazines about ladies who had previous c-section scars and had successful natural births. However, their scars were unlike mine. Since mine went up and down vertically, and my uterus had been cut open to remove the fibroid tumor, I was never allowed to go into labor for fear of rupturing and bleeding to death, so C-section births it was.

After my pregnancy with baby number one, I went back on birth control because my cycles began to worsen yet again. After a while, I began to have the horrible IBS stomach attacks. I assumed that something in my hormones while pregnant had allowed me the blessed reprieve, and now that my body was back to normal, my problems simply returned. My first child was two or three years old and was having to help care for mommy at times. She was such a little trooper, and never got scared by what she witnessed. She is now an amazing young woman by the way.

After several years dealing with flare ups from my IBS again, I also started having some strange skin issues, which in speaking to my sister yet again, found out it was Fibromyalgia. I would have areas on my body where it felt like a patch of cactus needles were stuck in my skin. Wearing pants or socks hurt as the friction against the affected area was very painful. There was nothing visible, only a patch about the size of a slice of bread. It would just suddenly come on, hurt for a few days to a week, then mysteriously disappear. This would happen about three to four times a year, usually in the same spot.

When my daughter was a newborn, I had to return to work, As I began a new job, I began experiencing something new one year, and for only that year. I started having these sudden bouts with my legs itching so badly after a shower that I would have to take Benadryl to stop it, making it impossible to go to work. Benadryl knocked me out. Even with all my weird ailments, I never missed much work. I was used to pain and sickness and just dealt with it. Except for the leg itching; that was relentless and life stopping and drove me utterly crazy. This too just stopped occurring for no reason, praise the Lord.

Years later, I decided that if we wanted to have kids again, I would have to stop the birth control pills. I soon got pregnant with my son and he was born when my eldest was four. About mid-way through my pregnancy with him, I contracted gestational diabetes and had to stay on a special diet for the safety of my baby as well as myself. I had to record every meal and a home health nurse would come to check on me once a week. Other than that, my pregnancy was uneventful. After he was born, my gestational diabetes went away as was expected.

About a year or two after my son's birth, we had the opportunity to adopt our youngest child. She was a special needs baby and would require a lot of extra attention. During this time of waiting, talking, and praying about this decision, my cycles became bad again and I had to go back on birth control to be able to function normally. The deciding factor here in my next

My Journey to Better Health

medical decision was the week where I spent three days on the couch and then could barely walk for the next four. Then, after only six weeks on birth control pills I realized that I started having severe IBS issues again. It then dawned on me that the pills changed my body so much that they caused my stomach issues to become severe. I related my story to my OB/GYN who stated that there was no way that was possible because the two issues were completely unrelated. Now, again, I'm no doctor, but even I knew then that the body works together in all things. So knowing this, I refused to take the pill, but I still needed something to help with menstrual pain. So, my doctor prescribed several different avenues for relief. We tried a vaginal insert, but that caused extreme burning that I could not tolerate. Again, I was told that was crazy and he had never heard of such a thing. Then he wanted to do an implant in my arm that would last for five years. I promptly said no. With the issues I had with everything else so far, I was sure I didn't want to surgically insert something that would have been difficult to remove should I experience issues with that as well. I then explained to my doctor that my only option was to have a hysterectomy because we were preparing to adopt a special needs child and I had to be able to care for that child. He was against my decision, citing all the problems that could arise from it, but I had no other options left. He thought I should just deal with the problems and not have the hysterectomy. But he had no idea how bad my cycles were and the life stopping pain they caused me. I can only assume he thought me to be a wimp and that I wanted an easy out. Another really good reason why we should never judge someone based on what we think we know. There is always more to a person's story than you know.

He did eventually concede to the surgery, and my only request was that he try to leave my ovaries if at all possible because it would lessen the effects of early onset menopause. This was not an option, however. During my procedure my husband had to make the decision to go ahead and remove my ovaries as well. My doctor explained that I had what was called oozing chocolate cysts on my ovaries and everything was basically cemented together inside due to that and the endometriosis. So, everything had to come out or else I would be back in a year having my ovaries removed anyway.

Again, I urge you to make your doctor listen to you. Only you know how you feel inside. No one else can tell you this, not even your physician.

For the first year after my surgery I felt amazing. I was losing weight, I felt great, no more painful cycles and my gut wasn't bothering me. I felt as though I had been given a new lease on life and I felt unstoppable.

It wasn't long however after that first year that I began to feel the effects of the surgery and inexplicably began to gain weight. I started having hot-flashes, exhaustion, my emotions were all over the place. I couldn't deal with stressful situations like I could before. And of course my IBS eventually reared its ugly head.

I would also crash around noon to two p.m. every single day. This in itself was frightening because I was home schooling my three children, and my youngest child's medical appointments were in Lafayette; which we

My Journey to Better Health

made monthly and was a two-hour ride in one direction. On those return drives home, I would get so sleepy while driving it was beyond frightening. This experience began my researching natural treatments, and my supplemental journey for the next ten years.

Chapter 2
The Next Twenty Years

God has had me in many different places in my health journey over the last forty years. And this has revealed to me many things about where I was at in life and what I had to do, or needed, to make my life function on a better level, even if that were only a temporary fix to get me through that period in time.

When the kids were young, I tried a weight loss program and was having success until the rules for the program changed. Their program no longer worked for me, but during that time I learned to like diet drinks over regular soda. I was a heavy soda drinker and attributed my weight gain to that. Unfortunately, switching to the diet drinks did not help with my weight. I tried different exercise programs, different diet programs, all of which did not help me. I had a hard time sticking to anything, because every time I started a new program I would gain weight; especially with exercise. Plus, having three children at home, all day, every day, truly limited my ability to do anything for myself. I just couldn't find the time to get away by myself. When my husband would come home from work, I didn't want to leave because I wanted to spend time with him. I was stuck in a rut which lasted for twenty-years. I still have trouble finding time for myself, even for appointments because my youngest is special

My Journey to Better Health

needs and can't be left alone for more than five or ten minutes.

So, this led to my weight gain along with constant running for school activities, eating while on the run, sitting during sports practices and games, and traveling all over the state of Louisiana for those games. However I noticed that most of the other mothers managed all of this without excessive weight gain. Why then did I struggle so much?

With all the new issues I was experiencing, I still had to deal with my gut issues. The female issues were now gone of course, but the severity of my IBS would come and go. Everywhere we went, I had to make certain to scope out where the restrooms were. I also had to take my special needs daughter along with me. Having to literally run to the restrooms, while trying to make a slow-moving child hurry up as well, was hard to manage.

Heat and cold affect my issues as well. I have learned over the years that if I start to cramp, if I can stay warm or hot, then the cramps will usually stop. This was especially hard in the summer when the temperature outside was one-hundred plus degrees and I would have to turn on the heat in the car just to make it home because I took a chill from cramping. I know this may sound strange to you, but my stomach starts to cramp, then I get goose bumps on my arms while I sweat at the same time from the pain, struggling to breathe because of the pain in my lower left side. For some strange unexplainable reason, extreme heat stops these symptoms.

To try to help some of my symptoms, I inquired at our local homeopathic store and started taking some supplements to help with adrenal fatigue for the afternoon tiredness. I also tried taking many other things to help with my IBS symptoms. I did learn from one of my sisters that my symptoms were relative to gluten allergy or intolerance. So, I started trying the whole gluten free thing. This I must say was hard to learn. It literally took me years to get it down and I still struggle with eating that way. I believe this is because of cooking for a family that is not gluten intolerant. I tried recipes they didn't like and therefore wouldn't eat. I had growing, active kids who needed nutrition so I gave up the gluten free lifestyle. I never noticed whether or not it actually helped because I never got to incorporate it long enough to see relief.

Later however, I did implement a gluten free way of eating, and it did help tremendously.

Another problem I used to suffer with was hip pain. It hurt while sitting or lying down and lasted for years. There were times that it hurt so badly that I couldn't sleep. Sometimes it would even bring me to tears. My husband, bless his heart, would massage my hips for me to alleviate the pain so I could rest. Yes, I have a wonderful husband. This was only a temporary fix though. I wasn't until after implementing the gluten free life-style completely that all of my hip pain simply vanished. I asked my chiropractor/nutritionist why this was, and he said that the intestines, if inflamed, will affect the surrounding tissues and nerves, causing pain in other areas. So, if you have hip or joint pain, try eating gluten free. And please, give yourself a few months of doing so to actually see if you can achieve results. A week or two might do it, but your body has to start to heal first.

My Journey to Better Health

As years went by the weight packed on, so I went to my general practitioner for help with weight loss, but the pills he prescribed were much too expensive. I then tried the over-the-counter weight loss plans but they did awful things to my gut. I also tried injections which did not work. I then asked my general practitioner at the time to check my thyroid as well as I was losing a lot of hair and my eyebrows were nearly gone, plus the feelings of tiredness, and crazy emotional swings. The tests revealed nothing and I was told my thyroid was fine. So I was back to square one.

Through the referral of a friend from church, I started seeing the chiropractor/nutritionist I mentioned just above, who ended up helping me through the roughest eight years of my adult life. Without this man and his wife, I don't know what I would have done. She would often sit and pray with a very emotional me over my issues as I sat in their waiting room, completely embarrassed at my uncontrollable crying problem. And he is a very compassionate man who listens to his patients. If not for them and how they handled their practice, I would likely have been on so many anti-depressant medications—like my mother and most of my sisters--and who knows what other types of medicines. He treated me for years with food-based supplements which helped immensely. I swallowed so many pills every day that it was depressing in itself. But I did it, because without those supplements I would not have made it through life at that stage. The only drawbacks to these supplements were the expense. They worked miracles with me, but they literally put us into debt. I would have to spend hundreds of dollars every month to purchase what I needed, on top of the office visits. But we did what we had to so that life for everyone could go on; my husband graciously stating that whatever I needed to function, we would do. As I got better, things would change. My body would change and certain products no longer worked for me. I truly even had some allergic reactions to some of the supplements, to the surprise of my chiropractor/nutritionist. I was an odd case to be certain. He couldn't understand how I could adversely react to some of these supplements. There was no reasoning for it, but he fortunately found another one that would work for me. He also informed me that I did indeed have a gluten intolerance and a thyroid issue.

Years passed with the ups and downs of supplemented life. I was still having gut problems, and menopause symptoms because of the complete hysterectomy. I continued to try to find more cost-effective ways to manage my crazy mood swings and hormone changes. I even tried the bio-identical, surgically-inserted pills for hormone imbalance. After two monthly insertions, these pills put me in such a high testosterone state that my entire body became fatigued and I could barely function. I then had to take a testosterone blocker to stop that from affecting me. It took months for my body to recover from that ordeal.

I promised earlier in the introduction, that I would expound further on God's grace in sparing me from cancer, so I will now begin that story.

Back in 2018, I believe, I had another strange occurrence happen. I was struggling with eating a full meal and barely ate a bird's portion of food. I would fill up quickly yet occasionally

My Journey to Better Health

gain weight. This went on for six months to a year. Then, I began to suddenly have upper back pain between my shoulder blades. I was also having tenderness in my upper abdomen area on both sides below each breast. The discomfort in my upper back began to grow until I was so uncomfortable nothing I did would ease the pain. After several days of this, I went to the doctor. I went to the local walk-in clinic and after the nurse-practitioner on call examined me and ran some minor tests, they could find nothing wrong with me other than some elevated enzymes. He then explained that would not cause the constant discomfort I was feeling, suggesting that with my history of IBS that I have a colonoscopy. He then referred me to have an MRI to see what could be causing the elevation in my enzymes and also gave me a referral to see a gastroenterologist.

The pain mysteriously went away after that and has never returned. If it has, it has been a very mild case of it. I do sometimes ache in my upper back, usually after much bending forward, but nothing like what sent me to the doctor before. After having an MRI to check my organs, they found that my spleen was slightly enlarged and my liver is covered with hemangiomas; little puffy blood vessels that stick up everywhere. They said they were harmless and would not have caused the back pain, just the tenderness I had experienced beneath each breast.. So, in the meantime, my gastroenterologist called to schedule the endoscopy and colonoscopy for even further testing.

A year prior to all of this, I was supposed to have a colonoscopy, but the doctor I had been referred to at that time wanted a large sum of money up front, which I didn't have so I gave up and forgot about the procedure. But God knew better and so here I was again, scheduled for the procedure once again.

The findings of those two tests were surprising. My stomach lining was slightly red and inflamed and so they tested me for Barrett's Esophagus, a possible cancer-causing disease of the throat. Fortunately the endoscopy test came back negative. I figured then that the redness in my stomach and lower esophagus was probably from the acid in the diet soda I drank regularly.

The colonoscopy however, revealed a few polyps, normally not a big deal; except that I had a massive one. One so large that every doctor and nurse I spoke with kept impressing upon me just how large it had been and that the doctor had to use two clips to close the hole on my intestine wall from its removal. I had to carry a medical alert card stating that I had metal in my body for a year after the procedure in case I was in an accident and they had to do an MRI. The tests on the massive polyp were not cancerous, yet. But the center was one step away from turning into cancer. I was told that if I had not had the procedure when I did, I likely would have been dealing with colon cancer in the very near future.

Once again, God's grace, provision, and intervention showed up in my life. I've seen His hand in my life so many times through-out my medical past. You see, if the pain had been in my gut area, I would have ignored it, as I was used to stomach issues, so going to the doctor for that would not have been an option. So, God gave me a strange pain elsewhere, one I had never before experienced to get my attention. If

My Journey to Better Health

not for that, my life may have taken on a different route.

After the procedure, my lack of eating ability ceased and I could eat an actual full meal, and the pains in my upper abdomen were gone as well. My last bloodwork report revealed that my enzymes were normal and my spleen had decreased in size. It's those realizations that God is always doing things for our benefit; even illness; that helps me to better take things in stride and to try to do better for my health.

On top of the ever-changing state of mind and body, I was now having issues with my teeth because of bone loss from the early onset of menopause due to my hysterectomy. To explain, let me give you some background on this.

When I was around nine or ten, I had two lower teeth pulled. I don't remember having pain, so I assumed they were baby teeth that would not fall out; the dentist back then pulling them to make room for my permanent teeth. Unfortunately, I did not have any teeth beneath the ones they pulled because nothing ever grew in. I never paid much attention to this because I never really had any issues with my teeth, until my early to mid-thirties. Now, as an adult with early menopause issues due to my surgery, my teeth began shifting. I now have a space in the front of my lower jaw where my teeth shifted backward filling in the gap where the baby teeth were removed. Yay me! Yes, I'm being sarcastic. Another one of my "conditions" from living life the way I have had to. You have to laugh sometimes or you'll go crazy.

By the way, I did however discover very recently from questioning my current dentist on that situation, that I have all of my teeth.

Meaning that the two teeth pulled when I was very young must have been extra teeth, so naturally, they removed them. Again, Yay Me!! Insert eyeroll here. Can you see it?

After years of continued IBS issues and constantly throwing up while at work, in town, at home, wherever my gut decided to throw a fit, my teeth did suffer for it. I did not have the wisdom, or someone else to inform me of the damage all that stomach acid running across my teeth at all hours of the day and night would do to them. I brushed when I was supposed to, but I did not have the foresight to carry a toothbrush with me at all times. Not that it would have mattered much. It wasn't like I had time to stop my job, dig through my purse, and go to the bathroom to brush my teeth every time my IBS would act up. I was a waitress and time moved quickly for me.

All of this also affected my social calendar more frequently than not. I would not or could not attend many events due to fear of my stomach acting up, or more than likely, the fact that it already was.

Friends we hadn't seen in years would be in town and I had to beg forgiveness for not visiting. My husband could go visit with them but I could not because I was sick with my gut. This ended up changing the way people interacted with me, I'm sure thinking that I just didn't want to be around them. I couldn't even attend my husband's class reunion with him. Why? Because my gut decided to act up that day. It always seemed to happen at the most inopportune times. This is the main reason why I won't commit to trying certain things. My husband has been after me to try scuba diving because he and my eldest daughter are both

My Journey to Better Health

certified. I would love to try it, but I won't take scuba diving lessons. It's cold beneath the surface of the water. The deeper you go, the colder it gets. When I get really cold, my stomach often decides to cramp. I can't afford to take that chance. So, unless I get rid of the cramping forever, I am limited on the things I can experience in life. Also, tight fitting clothing can also bring on an attack. Have you ever seen a loose-fitting wetsuit? Me neither.

It's rough at times, really. With menopause making me hotter than normal, and my stomach not liking the cold, finding a happy medium is difficult to say the least. But if I can control what goes into my system, then I have a better time of controlling how my body reacts to the stimuli.

Another side effect of my complete hysterectomy years ago is that I also deal with broken blood vessels in my face. The area on my cheeks, below my eyes, shows the stress of the twenty-year hormone battle. Sometimes these vessels are so dark that women have asked if I have written on myself with a pen. This was especially unnerving at times, especially since at one point I was known as the Dove girl in certain circles. Do you remember the Dove Soap commercials from twenty years back? When younger, I never wore makeup and I never had blemishes. That is no longer the case. I don't deal with acne much at all, but those blood vessels are a constant companion and do not clear up like a pimple will. I still don't wear much makeup though. I feel that if I have to cover up who I am, what's the point? So, I have learned to be comfortable in my own skin. No matter how marred it is now. But I don't have it so bad, especially when I see others who have much worse skin issues than I do, and I thank

God for his graciousness every time he brings someone worse off across my path.

Another thing that worries me about those visible spider veins is that my grandmother on my father's side had horrible varicose veins in her legs. I believe that is what eventually killed her, so I watch for this. I even sometimes feel or think I see a little puffiness in the ones in my cheeks. But then the next day, it seems they are small again. Now that that I am over fifty, I have been seeing broken vessels in my legs as well. They aren't varicose veins yet, and I hope they never become so, but it is a concern.

Now I am going to share with you something I discovered a few years back in 2019 when our church had a period of fasting. During this time, we were told to fast from whatever our current addictions were. We didn't have to give up everything, just what we craved the most. It didn't even need to be food related. Some gave up computers, social media, television; whatever had the biggest hold on us at that time. We were to fast from this for twenty-one days as this was the amount of time required to break a habit.

At that time in my life, my biggest addiction was diet drinks. One in particular, but I will not state which brand for legal purposes. Remember years earlier when I was told to switch to the diet drinks to help with my weight loss? Well, it didn't help. As a matter of fact, I now truly believe it was slowly killing me. I will elaborate more on this one topic in Chapter 5.

Now, I have had to return to some supplements, but nowhere near what I needed before. As I age, I still deal with things. At the moment that thing is still unexplained weight gain, diabetes, and have been diagnosed with

My Journey to Better Health

Hypothyroidism. Yes, even though I was told ten years ago that my thyroid was fine, it was not. One of the stranger symptoms of my thyroid disease was a pulling feeling in my throat, especially when strained. I used to sing a lot at church but had problems continuing this because of this pulling pain. Other times, my throat would feel like someone had their hand wrapped around it, squeezing. I wasn't choking at all, it just felt swollen, Because of my Hypothyroidism, my voice changed and I no longer sounded like I did when younger. Another reason to stop singing. I started treatment for this, but later discovered that I am unable to take thyroid medication because my body, again, has adverse reactions. I started having a medical problem called frozen shoulder. It is a common symptom of thyroid disease and diabetes, which I figure has more to do with the medication to treat these diseases. But don't take my word for it, do your own research.

It was then that I accidentally discovered that my thyroid medication was causing me severe joint pain after a recall on the semi-natural thyroid medicine that I was taking. I was placed on another medication and, shortly after, started to experience pain in my feet and ankles to the point where I could not walk. It was so bad that even when I was sitting, the searing pain would bring me to tears. Pain medications did not help to alleviate the pain. My shoulder was still aching and was now even worse. Then when I started to have hip pain as well on top of the shoulder and ankle pain, I began to get depressed again.

I haven't yet mentioned the depression I went through with all of the hormone changes and varying health issues. I never took medication for that as the supplements helped to manage it, but with all of the health issues over the years, my on again, off again, days of depression were never a surprise. I knew that my depression would be a constant with the lack of control over my own body and situation. It has changed my personality over the years. It is hard to truly be joyful and happy, and it is something I pray about. I know others who suffer from severe depression. Life can be hard, but it is much harder to handle without Jesus.

Anyhow, it seemed every time I started to do well physically; I would get knocked back down again. I pulled myself together and decided that this was no coincidence. I called my doctor and told them that the new thyroid medication was causing me very painful side effects and I was told to stop taking it. Unfortunately, there was not another brand for me to take. That was it. I had to figure something else out. That was when I found a product called Thyadine which I purchase from Amazon. It works wonders for my thyroid and doesn't seem to have any adverse effects for me. I pray it never does because it is the last option for thyroid care that I have been able to find.

God works in mysterious ways. Had it not been for that recall on my semi-natural thyroid medication, which I didn't realize at the time was also causing my shoulder pain, I would have never discovered my adverse reactions to the medication. You must be your own greatest advocate because only you know how your body reacts to things, and only you can make others stand up and take notice. Help your doctor help you by paying attention to your own body's reactions and taking the necessary

My Journey to Better Health
steps to learn from it, and don't let others tell you you're crazy, you're not. Special and different, maybe, but not crazy.

Chapter 3
Faith's Story

I remember my health challenges starting with lots of stomach problems when I was around the age of eleven. I was a very active, physical kid. For the most part you'd never know that I was sick, so it was hard for people to realize just how sick I could become. I dealt with lots of pain and throwing up. Mama spent a lot of time with me in emergency rooms and I too was told there wasn't anything wrong, I just wanted attention. Mama finally took me to a doctor when I was twelve and they did tests and x-rays, and determined I had a peptic ulcer. At the time, ulcers were associated with stress, so there was the concern that I wouldn't see the age of sixteen according to the doctor. But they were wrong and much later in my adult life I was treated for the bacteria that caused the ulcers. Papa had also had a long history of stomach problems, ulcers included, so it was determined that I took after Papa. Genetically speaking, I think it was inevitable. A few years later I had even more stomach issues from the scar tissue the ulcers caused. I can't begin to tell you all the barium I have consumed over the years for testing purposes.

As a kid who was hesitant to swallow medication, I always kept waiting for the milkshake they promised me, I even ask for it after the barium, but alas I never got it. For those of you who aren't aware, they told me the

My Journey to Better Health

barium was a milkshake so I would drink it. Now, I was not stupid and I knew that what they had given me was medicine for the test. But since they promised me the milkshake, I kept expecting them to bring me one because they had said they would. If you are unfortunate enough to have to deal with sick children in this manner, don't underestimate your kids intelligence. They are not stupid. Just explain to them, they usually will understand and appreciate not being lied to.

Anyway, to continue; the ulcerative scars were literally clogging up my duodenal area of the small intestines. My stomach became easily inflamed because of the bacteria, which had not been addressed yet, and I was not able to keep medicine down. As soon as it hit my stomach, I began throwing it back up.

As a kid I hated food. Some of the things mama would cook I would have to leave the house because of the smell turning my stomach. I'm still not overly fond of food. It has never been my friend with all my sensitivities and allergies.

We grew up in a house with about eight to ten people and only had one bathroom between all of us; mostly females too. Our oldest sister, Vanessa, and I had to take turns in the bathroom because we were constantly throwing up for one reason or another. Vanessa suffered from migraines back then and still does, even in her adult years. But my parent's determination in finding out what the problem was, managed to get me to a better state. I do not remember how, but I do remember being well enough to be able to play like the other children. Doctors had told them back then that I wasn't necessarily unhealthy, I just had a lot of medical issues.

Years later, when I started my monthly cycle at the age of fifteen I would become very sick with my stomach and had extreme pain with my menstrual cycles. They usually kept me in bed for a few days every month, and even affected my schooling as I had to often leave school because of the pain. At one point it became so frequent that my father even had to go talk to the principal because they did not believe that I was that sick. Later at the age of sixteen or seventeen I was diagnosed by a gynecologist with having endometriosis. This diagnosis finally explained why I was always so sick with my monthly cycles, and on top off my already peptic ridden stomach issues I missed a lot of school. Also around this time I began experiencing debilitating pain all through my body, but it primarily affected my neck, shoulders, and arms, but at most times also hurt the tops of my hips where they connected with the back. It never mattered what position I was in; standing, sitting, sleeping, using my arms, or not using them, the pain would not let up. Eventually, I went to see a muscle specialist to find out why I hurt all the time and was diagnosed with Fibromyalgia and Chronic Fatigue. There wasn't a lot known about these diseases back then and stress was the only known culprit at the time. Fortunately, nowadays, there is much more information from studies which point to food allergies as the cause of inflammation of the nerve endings. At that time though, all I could do was try to manage it with pain medications and anti-depressants.

Unfortunately, I wasn't able to tolerate the pain medications as it caused more stomach problems so they then gave me anti-anxiety

My Journey to Better Health

medicine to keep my stress levels under control. A *band-aid* fix that did not truly address the issue, but then, my doctors really did not know how to address the issue at the time.

The pain from the Fibromyalgia Syndrome was so bad that at times I had to put my right arm in a sling and I could not stand for anyone to touch my neck or shoulders; even to try and help by massaging the pain out. The simple act of being touched was more than I could stand. Over the years the severity of the pain would fluctuate and at times it became bearable, but the fatigue associated with the disease was my constant companion.

The renewal that sleep should have brought was not my friend, as I slept very poorly; which in turn just compounded my issues. This led to my stomach and digestive issues worsening, and I had to go see yet another specialist, a gastroenterologist. I was then diagnosed with Irritable Bowel Syndrome, but since my IBS symptoms were so severe I was checked out for Crohn's Disease, but luckily that test came back negative.

Some symptoms like constipation and diarrhea were constant companions. Eating takeout or in a restaurant was a challenge because the food would almost instantly begin to cause my stomach to roil as I rushed to find a bathroom. It was always difficult to determine what would or would not make me sick. At the time, my husband could not believe that food could move so quickly through my system until I proved it to him by showing him the barely undigested food in the commode. Apparently, some people take a lot to be convinced, but hey, he *needed* to know whether he was right or not, and since I am a people pleaser, I showed him just how wrong he was.

I eventually was able to control this somewhat by watching what I ate, staying away from rich foods and medications. Unfortunately I now cannot remember what kind of medicines had affected me adversely. Anti-anxiety meds were used mostly to control and relax my digestive system, and I remember a particular time where I was rushed to the hospital in an ambulance because we thought I was having a heart attack because of the terrible pain in my chest. That pain turned out to be a very deep ulcer in my duodenal channel which caused such strong spasms that the pain was felt in my chest. I was in so much pain that the ER doctor gave me a shot of muscle relaxer to help which worked. I was better afterward, except for the task of healing the ulcer which required a hospital stay.

My next health issue came about in the form of gallbladder disease. I want to say I was about twenty-six when I began to constantly experience sickness with lots of pain, throwing up, bloating, pressure, acid reflux, and other things. When I went to doctors for this, they just wanted to treat me for ulcers. I told them I had plenty of experience with ulcers and it did not feel the same. But they would not listen to me even though I was well versed on the subject. One doctor even went so far as to tell me that all I needed to do was get a job and get out of the house. GEESH.

I finally convinced a doctor to do an ultrasound and he found lots of gall stones in the gallbladder. There were so many that the technicians doing the ultrasound just stopped counting at thirty-five. I remember overhearing

My Journey to Better Health

them talking and was so relieved that someone had finally found something, because now they would have to listen to me and fix the problem. When they performed the surgery, they also found three stones embedded in my bile duct, and around fifty more stones in the gallbladder. The doctor told my husband I had to have been in terrible pain, confirming my complaints of pain all those years. That is always the biggest problem isn't it, getting other people to believe the intensity of the pain we experience. Living with pain had become normal, and so I learned to function regardless. Because I had dealt with the pain from having ulcers at the age of twelve I could manage and function when needed. My sisters and I always like to joke and say, "Mama and Papa didn't raise any wimps.".

The doctor performed the surgery to remove my gallbladder which required a seven-inch incision on my right side.

I remember back then hearing snide comments from girls regarding my scar when I wore a two-piece swimsuit to a lake beach. If they had only known the relief from pain that I felt. That scar did not bother me one bit, because it meant I was free from the debilitating sickness of gallbladder disease. People really do not have a clue sometimes about the important things in life. Scars tell stories about the things you have overcome. Don't let someone else's ignorance bother you. You my friends are overcomers, or hopefully will be one day very soon.

Throughout my health journey, one of the most annoying things I have dealt with was when people would look at me and tell me I looked fine, that I didn't look sick. These people were not with me all the time and they didn't see the times when I hurt so badly I couldn't get off the couch or have the ability for basic functions. There were times where I felt well enough and appeared perfectly fine where I could do what was needed, but then there were also times that my illnesses would suck the life right out of me. My uncontrollable illnesses would cause me to be left out of life's enjoyable moments quite often. Because I knew I was missing out on things, I would suck it up and make myself do stuff because I didn't want to be left out. Plus, I had a husband that expected my company on outings. Because I often pushed my body beyond its limits, I would end up being so exhausted that I would risk falling asleep when I drove. I remember vividly one such instance, while driving along a road I drove regularly, I literally could not recognize where I was and I truly had no idea; and that happened more than once. Looking back now, I cannot tell you how many times I can see where God has protected me.

Exodus 23:20 says:

> *"Behold, I am going to send an angel before you to guard you along the way and to bring you into the place which I have prepared."*

Thanks be to God for his provisions. For guardian angels and for preparing ahead for us. We are truly loved by a doting Father.

During my health issues, there were years where my illness prevented me from holding a job because I just could not function. During this unemployable period in my life I started having attacks that mimicked seizures. I would literally

My Journey to Better Health

turn into a limp noodle for thirty to forty-five minutes each time. I wouldn't pass out; but my body would become so weak that I could barely lift my arms. I would also experience involuntary jerking and twitching of my arms and legs. I couldn't even stand or sit up, and I could barely speak to where my words were slurred like I was drunk. One of these attacks came upon me once while driving and I had to pull off the road and wait for it to pass. After the attack, and I made it home, I was so weak all I could do was lay around for hours. I would also have anxiety attacks with these episodes that would further immobilize me.

Eventually, it was discovered to be yet another health issue that brought on these attacks. My heart was not getting the blood and oxygen that it needed to function properly. Many people who knew me, thought I was just having an emotional breakdown of some sort, but it was an actual, physical, medical problem that resulted in the side effect of anxiety. I found a teaching hospital called the Cleveland Clinic in the state of Ohio. I traveled there, hoping they would know what was now happening to me. They first tested me on a tilt table that mimicked my seizure like attacks. I had to lie flat on a table, and then they would raise me up to an upright position. This simple motion brought on my attacks; causing my heart to race, uncontrollable anxiety and crying, and such weakness afterward that I could not stand on my own. Further testing revealed the cause of these symptoms. I was diagnosed with two different diseases. One is known as Venus Pooling; a disease where blood gathers in the lower legs and cannot make the journey back up the body to the heart, thereby causing anxiety for the heart which then brings on a full-blown anxiety attack. The second is known as Hyper-Beta State Heart-where the heart gets confused about when it should beat fast. This testing showed that my heart would not beat fast when it needed to, but instead would beat fast when I was in a reclining or resting position. Through trial and error, I have since discovered that a potassium supplement helps me to regulate this problem with my heart.

I've also discovered throughout my life that my body reacts oppositely to what prescribed meds are supposed to do. This reaction could simply be the possibility that I have quickly built up a tolerance to them and they have simply stopped working.

As time went by and I began to learn to deal with these new illnesses I was also soon diagnosed with Autoimmune Deficiency Disease. This is not to be confused with AIDS. AIDD unlike AIDS is not that bad, thank God. It simply means that your body's immune system is off kilter. Instead of working for you, it is constantly fighting against itself, trying to heal your body, but this constant struggle within you only compounds your issues; the same issues that your medications are trying to fix. I believe that most of this happens because of the ill side effects that are always in abundance with mechanized medications. Adding to these problems is the other issues that can be caused by these medications, like fibromyalgia, chronic fatigue, food allergies—which I'll address later—and a myriad of other annoying problems. I learned early on that my body did much better on natural alternative medicines instead of the typical manufactured medications. I still had to deal with some side effects in the trial-and-error part of regulating these meds, but I did eventually manage to find the right supplements that actually helped my body.

Earlier I mentioned Venus Pooling and Hyper-Beta State Heart and I would like to give you a bit more information on the suggested medical fixes for these diseases. Other than suggesting salt tablets for the circulation issue of Venus Pooling, there was nothing offered to help with this issue. But, once I learned what was happening to my body, I then had the knowledge I needed to know what to do when I felt an attack coming on. I would lay flat on my back and raise my feet and legs above my head until I began to feel better. This was not an instructed practice by the doctor. This I figured out for myself based on what they told me was happening. Now, this simple act did not fix my problem, but it certainly made the symptoms from the attacks more manageable. Knowledge is power. If you learn what's happening within your own skin, and take action for yourself, you can find ways to help yourself deal with your illnesses. Don't wait for someone else to do it, because they truly do not know what you are feeling, only you do. Having said this, I do believe doctors are more knowledgeable than we are, and they have spent years in college and in medical training to discern your problems, but you can take the information they offer you and go even further from there, especially if they offer you no relief or only medications to help with the symptoms instead of fixing the problem.

Back to my two diagnoses. Because of the Venus Pooling and Hyper-Beta State Heart I found working to be very difficult, but I did manage it part-time with a company that was very lenient with me. Now, I still struggled with all these health issues and was continuously searching for a resolution. My doctors ran every test in the book from blood to diabetes testing. Every test came back "normal", no red flags of any sort of disease in my body. Fortunately, while working with this company, I discovered a doctor through word of mouth that worked very hard to discover *why* people were sick instead of just treating their symptoms. This physician was a vascular surgeon who carried on the tradition of holistic medicine from his father, who had also been a doctor. This was a sort of side business for him.

On my first consultation with him, he told me all the things he believed was going on in my body, which he followed up with testing to confirm his thoughts. He informed me of the labs he would use, why he trusted them, and then showed me all the test results and discussed them all with me. He also gave me all the information on the labs so I could verify for myself their authenticity. He then explained the treatment procedures, most of which used holistic medications, and the reasons he chose those particular ones. He also was not against the use of antibiotics and other medicines as necessity required.

His findings for my problems and symptoms were as follows. The first findings being Lyme disease which he thought came about from a vaccination I had received right before it was removed from the public because it was infecting people; possibly those of us with immune compromised health like me. This was further enforced by the fact that my husband also took the vaccine and did not have the same issues that I did. Having said this, he also never had a Lyme disease test performed. Next on the list was metal poisoning including lead, mercury, and arsenic metal. There were others that I can't recall, but the levels in the three mentioned above were way too high for the body to handle.

The lead was kind of obvious growing up in the era in which I did, where lead paint was prevalent, as well as the source of the mercury. Papa had worked in the coal mines, so coal dust and a coal heated house was the obvious cause for the mercury poisoning. Not to mention that people don't realize that there is a process in treating coal using mercury; the next highly listed poison in my body. There is also mercury in our silver fillings, or there used to be. Amazing isn't it? Last but not least is the arsenic metal which is a naturally occurring element in ground water – more commonly found in deep water-wells. We grew up drinking well water and this continued into my adult years as well. Our wonderful, clean-tasting well water had high levels of arsenic metal. After this information was given to me, I had it tested and both labs gave the same results. Because of this I chose not to have a third lab test the water, I was convinced with the same two results from the previous tests.

I was also diagnosed with having a gluten allergy which would attest to the extreme issues I continued to experience. Things the other medicines and health fixes had not taken care of.

A fun side note for you here: After learning that I had gluten allergies, I then went to my gastroenterologist and ask him to run tests to confirm this diagnosis so he could advise me how to further handle this issue. The man actually said, "that it was not a good idea to have that confirmed or have a test done, because it was so difficult to live gluten free, and it would be too hard for me to deal with." Really? I was flabbergasted! And I told him so. Why would this man advise me against something to help me learn more about this disease so that I could actually get better? I can only assume that at the time there was so little known about gluten allergies that he thought it was a *lifestyle choice* and not a *real health concern*.

Proverbs 24:6 says:

> *For by wise guidance you will wage war, and in abundance of counselors there is victory.*

Proverbs 1:5 tells us:

> *A wise man will hear and increase in learning, and a man of understanding will acquire wise counsel.*

The Bible warns us about listening to the wrong people. Seek wise counsel. Now a doctor is wise counsel, but they may not always go that extra step or mile to do what needs doing. Keep looking for that one doctor that will.

OH MY GOODNESS! I was truly sick, and I told him just how sick I was, and the man had been treating me for being sick. Why wouldn't he, as my trusted doctor, want to help me figure this out? By this point I was losing all respect for doctors. Yep! Especially since the gluten that my intestines could not digest caused the filter hairs in the intestinal tract—those hairs that filter out nutrients from the food you eat to sustain and nourish your body—to die because I could not digest the gluten! That sounded like a good reason to me to look into this further and to find a way to survive this digestive onslaught. When you take it upon yourself to do the research, you also find out lots of other aches and pains the body can go through because of inflammation caused by a gluten allergy.

Let's go back to the treatment process by the physician who found my underlying issues. First, I underwent intravenous Chelation Therapy to remove the heavy metals from my body. This treatment was first used for workers in automobile factories for pulling the poisons in paint that got trapped in the body. I had also begun taking the necessary antibiotics for the Lyme disease. My tests registered a high level of the antibodies due to the parasites in my system. Because of the damage to my nervous system, it was not repairable, but we could stop further damage.

The process for fixing my gluten allergy was of course food related. I had to stop eating anything that had wheat or grains in it or that were processed or contaminated by wheat and grains. This covers a lot of stuff!! Wheat primarily is white processed flour, but there are also grains and other flours you would have never thought of until you had to know. This has been a process covering years, but I can attest to the proof in the pudding, so to speak. I did, and still do, have proven results from my gluten free diet. It truly works, but it is so expensive.

Now, I love bread, but gluten free bread is *not* like wheat bread. I miss bread, but I *loved* feeling better more than I loved wheat bread, so I managed. Now-a-days, things have come a long way since I first started my gluten free journey many years ago. Palatable bread is mush easier to find out there. The primary principle of eating gluten free is this; if you keep it simple and prepare your food yourself, you can control your diet. When you go out to a restaurant, gluten free is now recognized, and you can tell your server that you must have gluten free. Don't be afraid to ask them, your health is important. Just be polite and try to keep your requests simple, it will work out. But when in doubt about what you are looking at or are unsure if it really is gluten free, just don't go there. It's not worth the sickness you will surely experience the next day or two.

Between the intravenous chelation, Lyme disease treatments, and the gluten free diet I did get better; better than I had been for a very long time. I was even able to resume working, which I did enjoy once I was not so deathly ill. But this was not the end of my health discoveries. I later found another gastroenterologist to help with my ongoing digestive issues. She was versed on the gluten allergy problems and made sure I did not have Celiac disease and guided me in the treatments for the gluten issues. Upon further testing I was then diagnosed with Gastro Paresis. A disease of the stomach that slows down the muscular contractions that digest food in the stomach, and then move it through to the intestines. In this discovery they also found a dark spot on my liver, but yearly testing showed no growth or change, so my doctor said it was most likely a bruise caused from the

My Journey to Better Health

gallbladder issues. My Gastro Paresis has proven to be another great hurdle to handle. Since my stomach does not empty well, it feels extremely full and very uncomfortable most of the time and a lot of foods are very hard to digest. I have learned to stay away from cow's milk because of the casein A. It causes extreme bloating and discomfort. I have replaced cow's milk with goat's milk mixed with unsweetened coconut milk. I do not use almond milk because it is nut based and has a lot of lectins. The combination of the two milks gives me a milk very close in taste to cow's milk. If this seems hard to understand, there is a process for American cow's milk that is different from European cows that can make a difference here; making products from European cows more tolerable; but do the research for yourself as it is too difficult to explain here.

During researching lectins, I have also discovered that lectins can have a negative impact on gluten intolerant people. This research has given me some very real results from limiting my lectins. You cannot be completely lectin free as it is in everything, but limiting lectins has been very helpful for my digestive comfort.

Now I'll explain more on my Gastro Paresis diagnosis. Oils, fats, veggies, beef, and other normally hard to digest foods, should be avoided. Eat small meals that can satisfy you, but not fill you up too fast. Liquid diets can also be helpful here. Also, getting plenty of physical activity will also make your system work better. Again I reiterate, research and paying attention to your system is key here. Knowledge is power and understanding how other people deal with their issues is helpful. Lots of research and trusted websites is important. There are a lot of dairy free products out there that make this easier for me. Again, you can learn to tolerate things when you have to. Your taste buds can adapt when you give them a chance.

Years ago, after a routine endoscopy by my doctor, she told me that she did not find any signs of celiac in my duodenal exam and it was possible to be free of my allergy after a five-year period of gluten free living. I was elated and ate wheat bread like a person who has experienced starvation! Boy was that a mistake! That bread made me so sick that I had extreme diarrhea for five weeks. Yep, you read that correctly. When I went back to her to see why I was so sick, she told me it was possible that I simply could not tolerate gluten regardless of the test not showing any more issues. I proceeded to ask her why she didn't tell me that instead of letting me think I was cured of the gluten allergy. Again, another hard lesson learned for your benefit. Don't jump back on the bandwagon to quickly after being given a clean bill of health. You may pay for it later. Take your time, and make sure the person giving you the information is correct.

To close out this lengthy journey regarding my health challenges, like my sissy Shawna, and my other sissies, as she has stated, we are all special and different in how our bodies deal with stuff. We do not fit the normal in the statistics. If that is you too, take heart. God knows all about you. I am better now than I have ever been. None of which would have occurred if God's hand of power and love were not directing me the entire way.

My Journey to Better Health

Isaiah 58:11 says:

> "And the Lord will continually guide you, and satisfy your desire in scorched places, and give strength to your bones; and you will be like a watered garden, and like a spring of water whose waters do not fail."

Again, He guides us in all things, we just must learn to recognize that when we feel alone, He is there with us, giving strength to our very bones, So trudge forth knowing He's got you.

I was led to each discovery through the prompting of my loving Father. I was able to see it then, and more so now, because we have an ongoing conversation. I have reached a better understanding of this as I grew older and wiser, and my relationship with God, Jesus, and the Holy Spirit has increased. Never attempt life without them or other godly people in your life. God can use ungodly people in your life too, but the godly ones are the ones you should gravitate to for help.

One of the supplements/foods I recently found to be very beneficial for me is celery juice from a juicing machine. Celery Juice is used for detoxing and for helping the liver to function more efficiently. It also helps tremendously with inflammation. The benefits I've found to be most helpful is in the energy department as well as inflammation and pain. I swear to you; it is like the elixir of life. I drink eight to sixteen ounces first thing in the morning on an empty stomach and do not eat anything for thirty minutes. I feel energized the entire day and the pain that I still experience in my hips diminishes so much. I'm sure the rest of my body benefits as well, but I noticed it mostly in my hips. However, not all celery is created equally. Find a store that has a good brand you like. I have found that if it is really green on the outside and reminds me of a green, sunburned potato, the celery has a very bitter taste. So, be careful when choosing your celery. To prepare mine for juicing, I use a potato peeler to shave off the outside skin and remove the leaves. This makes it much more palatable. I tell you this to encourage you in your attempts. Don't give up after your first try, give it a few more chances because it has been so very helpful to me.

I do still struggle with health issues, but I shudder to think where I might be without all of the improvements that I have experienced over the years. God has truly been so very gracious to me, and I am grateful for his leading in more ways than just my physical health.

Isaiah 42:16 tells us:

> *I will lead the blind by a way they do not know. In paths they do not know I will guide them. I will make darkness into light before them, and rugged places into plains. These are the things I will do, and I will not leave them undone.*

He has certainly led me over the years and turned my many dark places to light. Praise be to His mercies and grace in my ignorance. Amen

My Journey to Better Health

Chapter 4
People

Without other people in our lives, we can't always see where God is leading us. It is through others and their experiences that we learn things that will help us. I know that when I feel poorly, I have a tendency to want to stay to myself; which is not really a good thing to do. We are meant to have people in our lives. We learn from others whether we realize it or not.

Now, I come from a large family. I am one of seven born siblings. I have come to learn over the years that many health issues are prevalent in our family line. My father's side of the family also boasts a large family of twelve siblings, half of which were girls. We, meaning my female siblings, have inherited the female issues from our father's side. My mother never really had any female reproductive problems. There is only one boy in our sibling group of seven, and he of course never had any health issues growing up. However, my sisters and I have. Not everyone had issues when they were younger, and every family goes through health issues at some point, but out of all of us, I and one of my eldest sisters, Faith, have had more issues than the others at younger ages.

You've read some of her story in the last chapter, but she was also born at home as my grandmother helped our mother deliver her.

My Journey to Better Health

Faith was born blue with the umbilical cord wrapped around her neck. My dad sat with her and unwrapped that cord, and thank God, she lived. That is how she got her name by the way. She battles with things on a daily basis now, but she handles them extremely well and her body now functions as a whole. She is capable of doing much more now in her older age than she could before. You see, she learned to pay attention to what her body told her, and daily takes the necessary steps to improve her situation, often choosing natural aids to help her body. I aspire to one day be as grown up as she is. Love you Faith. You are my inspiration in so many ways.

Okay, enough of the mushy stuff. Anyway, with her guidance throughout the years with some of my health issues, I came to learn that we were very similar in some areas. I also am like my other sisters in other health areas. Being the baby, I apparently got the lion's share of the physical problems. I was both blessed and cursed to have a little of everything everyone else had. Oh well, if that is what God wanted then who was I to argue about what He gave me to deal with. Having said this, my life isn't so bad really. I do struggle with things more now, but a lot of my current issues are my own fault from lack of attention to myself over the years. I put my family first in all things, thereby neglecting myself; shame on me. We mama's must learn to care for ourselves too. It truly was unconsciously done. Running for sports, school, life in general. Grabbing whatever we could because we were starving, and still had hours before we would make it home, or I was so worn out that I just couldn't fathom cooking at eight or nine at night. You see, we ran more than the average family because I homeschooled our children. I was responsible for their education in all areas. We didn't have a set location at which to play sports or to learn music. I had to take them out wherever our homeschool group was allowed to meet, or find extracurricular programs for them to do, such as music, art, social clubs, 4H, etc. Now due to this constant running, and mostly sitting on my part, my physical abilities slipped little by little over the years, and the weight packed on slowly. I did try several different options to control my weight with little success. I think my body's very "different chemical makeup" for lack of a better description, may have something to do with my inability to succeed with most programs geared toward the normal human being. Anyway, now you already know my story. But what you don't know is that by speaking to others around me and in my life, I have discovered better ways of dealing with my issues. I discovered many of the things that I now use to help my body just in conversing with others..

It was in speaking to a neighbor and friend that, I found my most recent God-send, Thyadine that I mentioned earlier. You see, my prayer life can get pretty intense at times. Having so many different health issues over the years tends to make one talk to God a lot. Can I still work on my prayer life? Absolutely. I still don't communicate with God as much as I should, but I have cried on his shoulder many, many times over the course of the last forty or so years. And through those tearful prayers often came the answers, although, I didn't always recognize them as such at the time. It is

My Journey to Better Health

upon reflection that I notice where God has worked. He has shown me many things about myself and others, as long as I was willing to look unbiased at those answers.

My neighbor friend's family was spread out the Thanksgiving of 2019 and she didn't feel like cooking for just herself and her youngest, so they asked if they could spend Thanksgiving with us. Little did I know that this simple request was an answer to my prayers. You see my friend has a decent sized family, and she usually cooked Thanksgiving dinner for them. Her parents are both still living, and she has siblings who visit from out of town. Plus she has three children and a husband, and many now older foster children who still visit them. But this particular year, it was only to be the two of them; my goodness how God works things out for our good. Had it not been for her visit that day, and my willingness to talk about my messy health issues, I may have never discovered Thyadine. She had used it for some symptoms of thyroid issues for a time, and happily recommended it to me to try.

Listen, I get it; people are messy. Life with people is messy. But life without people would be unbearable. If not for the wisdom of others, and the trials and tribulations that they have gone through, we wouldn't be able to learn how to traverse our own trials and issues. Sure, we might be able to figure things out eventually. But isn't it so much easier to learn from those who have already experienced the very things we are currently struggling with? Just the simple act of speaking to a fellow human being can greatly affect our own lives. Therefore, the reason for this book.

The Bible often speaks of the power of the tongue.

Proverbs 18:21 says:

> *The tongue has the power of life and death, and those who love it will eat its fruit.*

Use your words for good and uplift others. Don't be afraid to share your own experiences and struggles with those who may be going through the same things. If you can't sympathize, then pray with them. You never know how your story will affect someone else's life. Being open and transparent isn't a weakness, it becomes our strength. You don't always have to pretend that you have it all together. Being vulnerable can be your greatest gift toward recovery, either for yourself, or for the next person who ventures across your path.

For many years I only spoke to my sisters a few times a year. Not because of any feuds or disagreements, simply because we all lived so far apart and had our own busy lives.

With the advancement of technology, we now not only get to speak to each other daily, we also get to see one another's faces through a communication app on our cellular phones.

This has been the greatest God-send of all. We are so much closer now. Most of us, not all-some can't handle the constant ping of notifications-speak almost daily, and in this, help one another deal with whatever life is throwing at us. We are so much closer now. We used to feel cut off from everyone because we hardly ever spoke or visited one another. Now we hardly miss a single day of interaction. We are a part of each other's lives, and therefore can wisely advise one another on all manner of life's trials and tribulations, and fully celebrate one another's joys and accomplishments. Again I say; life is messy and people are messy, but oh what a mess! We can all make a mess together, and even share a laugh over it now and again.

Staying connected to one another is easier than it ever has been before. But most of the time, we spend it looking at junk, reading about the lives of people we don't know, or trying to keep up with people on our social media accounts. I very rarely post anything about my family on my social media accounts. I don't because I tell them in person or in other ways what they mean to me. I don't need to tell the world, only the ones it truly matters to. My husband, children, and family know I love them through personal interaction with them and them alone. I need no one else's approval.

Chapter 5
Levels of Health

I believe there are differentiating levels of health. Not everyone can be at the same level. You only need to aspire to be better than you were yesterday; to take the next step to improve your health. Don't try to do what the healthier person next to you can do. Accomplish what your body is capable of doing without hurting yourself and being down and out for the next week or more. And don't worry about what that person next to you, behind you, across the room from you, thinks or says. They don't know your whole story or how your body reacts to things. Only you truly know what happens beneath your own skin. You don't need to try to impress anyone; you just need to try to get healthier for you and your loved ones. Manage what you can, and when you feel ready to push yourself a bit more, then take that next step.

I am currently in a much better place than I was even a year ago; fit for my current stage in life. Am I in top physical condition at my current age? No, I am not, but I am finding *my* healthier level for *my* stage of life. I am trying to improve myself at the pace in which I can manage. Getting healthier is a constant state of work, but aren't most things?

According to most of my blood work numbers and reports, I *am in* good health. Of

My Journey to Better Health

course I do have some issues that have crept up, like diabetes, which I am trying to control without medication because, as you already know, most medications do not agree with me. But if I do not get it under control soon, I may have to give medicine a try, as much as I dread the thought of it.

Now, exercise is something I am trying to do more. I notice that I do feel so much better with even a small level of activity. This is a continuous work in progress as well. Being a writer makes it even more difficult as I do a lot of sitting, so I must be more mindful to get exercise into my daily routine.

I try to walk early in the mornings since it is really the only time I can find to do so. My sisters and I have discovered that we *must* exercise to lose weight, and more often than not, it is a sweaty, bent over, breathing hard, and near passing out, physical kind of exercise. Our hearts have to get pumping or else our body types just hold onto the fat, like a bear storing it up for winter hibernation. We will seldom dehydrate or feel hungry, because our bodies are storing so much of our own fat. Then, we must deal with weight gain before weight loss as our bodies pack on the muscle before burning off the fat. Every time I start an exercise program I will gain weight. It can be very frustrating at times. I just have to remind myself that muscle weighs more than fat, and I still have muscle memory from being an active young adult.

Exercise should be easier for me because I have many things at home to aid in this. Do I use them all? No. Should I? Yes. We are fortunate enough to have an above ground pool. We have almost always had one for the kids. Now, it is round and mainly for playing or just floating in, and I like to swim when I get into the water, and you can't exactly swim well in a round twenty-two-foot pool. Fortunately, I have found these awesome swim bands that hook to the poolside which allows me to swim for as long as I wish in a stationary position. Yes, they cost a little money, but if you can't spend a little of what you earn on your health, then what good is earning the money in the first place? Trust me, I too felt guilty spending money on myself, especially when the kids were young and it was a struggle to make ends meet, but I am past that stage in life and choose to spend a little on myself. It took me years to get to this mindset. You are just as important as everyone else in your household. More so, because without you, things would likely fall apart. Am I right? Take care of yourselves, so that you can take care of your family. And this goes for you dads as well. You are likely the breadwinner for the family. You are important to your family. Take the time to exercise, even if it is just a walk around the neighborhood. Take a walk with your wife and kids. It can be a great bonding time, and you are teaching them good habits as well. Now I'm not saying moms can't be the breadwinners too. I know that in this day and age, many are, but if you are also working and fulfilling all the mama chores too, then you definitely need to learn to relax and take care of yourself. And exercise is an awesome way to do this. You sleep better, feel better, and it releases stress in the body and the mind. You are worth it.

Find something you like doing. In today's world, there are so many things right at your fingertips. You can live stream dancing weight

My Journey to Better Health

loss programs. There are workouts with minimal to no added accessories needed and little space required. Even try playing one of the gaming systems with your kids. Most households have one of these devices nowadays. If you think they are just for kids only then you my friend are missing out on great fun, and exercise in the process. Especially the dance games for some of these devices. My kids always have a blast doing these, and I have a blast watching them, but participating is even better. Show those kids we were once kids too with your awesome dance moves from back in the day. It is always better to find something you enjoy doing because you are more likely to make the time to do it. And with the world at your fingertips, searching for something you enjoy, and that is possible to do where you live, wherever that is, is an easy target to manage. You used to enjoy your life as a kid, get that feeling back and find something to enjoy now; whatever that might look like for you. Health isn't just physical. It's a mental, emotional, and spiritual journey that affects every aspect of our lives. If you are uncertain about what that looks like for yourself then pray about your journey and let God lead you.

Jeremiah 29:11 talks about this:

> *For I know the plans I have for you," declares the Lord. "Plans to prosper you and not to harm you. Plans to give you hope and a future."*

He has a plan for your life, and part of that plan is He wants you to be happy, and the sooner you get on the same page as God, the better you'll feel. You might not have an easy time of it because Satan doesn't want you fulfilling your God given goals for your life. He wants you down and out. He wants you to question whether you are really doing the things you should. He wants you discouraged and giving up. He wants to steal your happiness, assuredness, and faithfulness. Don't let him have any of it. God created you for something wonderful. You have a purpose.

Ephesians 1:11 tells us:

> *Before we were even born, he gave us our destiny; that we would fulfill the plan of God who always accomplishes every purpose and plan in his heart.*

Meaning, God doesn't make mistakes. You are not accidentally here on this earth, no matter what others may tell you. Ask God to show you what His purpose for you is and follow through. No matter how hard it gets; God led you to it, and He will see you through it.

My Journey to Better Health

Chapter 6
Trying New Things

Many things can have an impression on us. We often allow those impressions to affect us in some way, whether it is good or bad. Often times, it is the way we think others will see us or worry about what someone else may think. The bible says in:

Proverbs 29:25:

> *It is dangerous to be concerned with what others think of you, but if you trust the Lord, you are safe.*

Does this mean you can do whatever you want regardless of what others think? No. Read the verse again. It states that if you trust the Lord, meaning that if you follow His teachings, you are safe. Be bold in what the Lord calls you to, not what you call yourself to. Don't interpret the Bible to suit your own needs or wishes but follow the teachings boldly.

Satan will tell us lies, and then we believe and allow those lies to take root. Lies and misconceptions often rule our thoughts and actions. Even the smallest ones, such as, I have no time for me. The more we tell ourselves these lies, the more they become habit. We often *have* the time, but we just don't *make* the time. We

My Journey to Better Health

tend to use it in other ways or make excuses, no matter how real those excuses are.

If we chose to, we could find time to do something for ourselves; something to aid us in our healthy pursuit; even if that decision was to eat healthier.

Instead of that candy bar, snack cake, or bag of chips, make a cake in a mug. Yes, it requires a little more effort -two minutes max including cook time- but it is worth it, is much healthier, and, in my opinion, tastes great. Having emphatically bestowed upon you the merits of 'cake in a mug' and the taste, please note that anything new that you try will likely taste odd or strange the first time as your body adjusts to the different ingredients. After that first one though, things begin to taste different, so don't give up. I have made things and hated them the first time, even though others praised the recipe. After returning a second time to try it once more, I enjoyed it so much I couldn't figure out what I had done wrong the first time around.

You can search for recipes that you might like, there are many different, healthy ones out there. I first heard of cake in a mug through the *Trim Healthy Mama* food plan, and I still use many of their recipes to this day. I also need to get back on the THM plan wagon again to aid in healthier eating and weight loss. Just another example of a good program I let slip away because of children's complaints over some of the meals.

I know, I know; be strong and do what needs doing. Insert another eyeroll here—at myself.

Some fights just aren't worth it, so I picked my battles back then. But now that my children are older and moved out, I can get back to a healthier way of eating.

That was something else I had to get used to; the way different foods tasted. Remember earlier when I said that I did not like diet drinks, couldn't stand them actually, but I willed myself to get used to them; only one brand in particular. My point here is we can get used to things if we wish to badly enough.

Now when I say I was a soda drinker, I mean it. I used to drink way too much; up to a twelve pack a day without even realizing it at times. I was always moving and doing things. Running here or there, busy and needing energy and sodas were an easy, flavor-filled grab. For years I drank them without worry because I thought they weren't affecting me in a negative way. Then, years later, I started seeing all the reports about the negativity of diet sodas. But, then every few years a report would come out about the negativity of some food or another. This was a reoccurring pattern in the scientific and media world for many years, and many reports were incorrect. So, I continued drinking my diet sodas, until the fasting for church was introduced.

Our pastor preached a sermon from the Bible about when and how to make things become a habit, and he had found that it usually held at or after a twenty-one-day period. We, as a congregation, were to give up whatever thing was our biggest crutch or vise. We were to abstain from our bad habits for twenty-one days. This challenge began my wellness journey and the way I found out just what it is that my body truly needed and what it did not need. Fasting for twenty-one days has been one of the greatest gifts that God has given me, medically.

My Journey to Better Health

I managed the fasting relatively easily and did not return to the diet soda afterward. I didn't drink soda for about a year or so after. And let me tell you the amazing thing that happened. For the first time in nearly ten years, my body began to level out. I no longer needed all the supplemental food nutrition pills, which helped immensely financially. I began to feel great, physically. I had energy, strength, my mental clarity was better, my emotions were more controllable, and my IBS issues got better; even though I had not been a diet soda drinker all my life. It dawned on me one day that I had slowly been killing my body over the years, simply by drinking diet soda. I truly believe that it was the great evil that kept throwing my body into complete and utter chaos. So, I say this in hopes that if you are an avid diet soda drinker, and have health issues, some very unexplainable, stop drinking the diet soda. It has truly made a huge difference in my life health wise.

Now, I had already been trying many new healthy options as you have previously read. And some worked for a while, but none have truly stuck. There are parts here and there that for the most part will still work for me. And I implement them as often as I can, but life seems to always interfere doesn't it? However, tomorrow is another day to start over fresh. Just continue to start each new day with a way to stick to your plans or try something new. Take what works for you and build your own plan. I know those bad habits are hard to break, and new good ones are hard to make. But I have found that repetitiveness, no matter how long it takes, generally wins out.

I am hard-headed, I'll freely admit to that. And because of it, I can have a hard time doing what I need to do. It can take me years to get the hang of something. But once I do, I usually stick to it. I'm not afraid of change, but I like the comfort of familiarity as much as the next person.

It's strange to say it can take me years to learn a new habit because I am constantly learning something new in life. I like a challenge and I'm not afraid to try new things or attempt to learn a new skill. I do however have my limits on this.

I refuse to jump out of a perfectly good airplane. I have a friend who is fulfilling her bucket list and parachuting was on the list. As much as I love her and support whatever it is she wants to do, I did not jump with her. Her bucket list is not my bucket list. And your friend's bucket list might not be the same as yours. However, if there is something that you have wanted to do, or see, or experience, then try to make it happen. Life is full of experiences and opportunities, so why not live and make some of your own that you would truly enjoy.

My husband has a bucket list and we have been fulfilling some of those for him. His and mine are not the same either. We have some things that are similar but not the same. I do try to participate in his since our lives walk the same path. What someone else wants to do may not be your idea of fun but walking the journey with them, tagging along for the ride, can be just as rewarding. Plus you never know when you might discover something else you enjoy.

My Journey to Better Health

Chapter 7
Paying Attention

One of the greatest things I've learned to do is pay attention to my body and how it reacts to things. What I eat, what I wear, what I put on my skin and hair, and the supplements and medicines I take all affect my health in some way. Yes, even certain types of clothing. If it isn't comfortable it's gone.

Do I always get it right? Nope! Sometimes I just crave that carb-laden, starchy, sugary, thing. I know I'm going to pay for it later, but at the time it so feels worth it. But alas, it usually is not. And I can't say that I've figured out a cure-all for those unquenchable cravings that drive you crazy. You know the ones I'm talking about. The ones where you eat everything in sight thinking this one will satisfy that craving, but nothing does. Then you spend the evening physically feeling horrible and possibly into the next day or even longer. And sometimes it is as simple as your body telling you that it is thirsty, and you just need some hydration.

Eventually you get to a place where you're tired of feeling sick and dealing with the consequences of poor decisions. That is where lasting change comes from. When you truly recognize the things that are making you ill, and are really ready for a change, then the possibilities begin to take shape.

I have accepted where I am for now. My body doesn't seem to crash as much as it used to. And it isn't on a roller coaster of physical and emotional ups and downs. I've finally figured out how to keep it running relatively smoothly. I have a few supplements that I use that work for me and I refuse to try any of the new things out there that promise energy, weight-loss, health, or whatever else. It took me a long time to get to this point in life where I can manage life without too many interruptions. I'm not about to mess it all up trying to shed these too many extra pounds. I will however do the next best thing and try to exercise more and be more mindful of what I eat.

I recently lost an immense amount of weight, thinking it was the Thyadine which afforded this wonderful change. But I soon realized that it was immensely high blood sugar levels which caused the weight loss. What!? I had always heard that glucose intolerance caused weight gain, and I have that in abundance. Although the Thyadine is a wonderful addition for my thyroid issues, alas, it was not the hero I once thought.

I discovered my highly elevated sugar levels due to a lingering, incapacitating, painfully life changing, yeast infection.

At the time I was eating a lot of carbohydrates and excess sugars. I wasn't having the usual IBS issues I used to have with the gluten, and I was dropping one to three pounds a week. I was active, feeling wonderful, and so excited to finally being able to shed all the extra pounds. Now, I knew I had high blood sugar issues, but I thought they were under control since I was losing weight so rapidly. Then, the yeast infection hit. At first I thought it was a bladder infection. After several trips to the doctor and several rounds of antibiotics because it would not clear up, I realized it was due to high blood sugar. I abruptly started watching what I was eating, and the infection cleared up. As my blood sugar went down, so did the weight loss. I am still working on my blood sugar levels as naturally as I can without medication, but I have begun to slowly regain some of the weight I lost. I know it is partly because of my diet, even though I am not eating badly; I just have to tweak what I eat and when and get back to being more mindful to exercise. Remember me, the body that holds on to fat like a bear storing it up for winter? So again, today is another day and I will choose better options for myself and try not to beat myself up if I make a bad decision. I also need to implement more of the things that worked for me before I got lazy and thought I could actually eat what I wanted. I will try to choose to do better for me and my family today. Will I fall again? Probably. But I will start again too.

My Journey to Better Health

Chapter 8
Being Consistent

Consistency is a hard thing to do. Trust me, I get that. But consistency does not have to mean daily, structurally, at all times, never unwavering. It simply means to get back to it eventually, but sooner rather than later. I know how easy good habits are to break and how easy bad habits are to fall back into. But, I have found over the years that the more we get back on track after falling off the proverbial wagon, the better chance we have of cementing that good habit in the place of that bad one.

I am a very long study of new habits. As I said before, I am a hard-headed person. This causes me to take long periods of time to learn something new, especially something good for me. An example is the years; yes years; it took me to get the gluten free way of eating down. And I managed to eat that way for years afterward. Do I still stick to that strict diet? No, but if I had to go back to eating gluten free again, it would be easier because I have already learned the skill and know that I am capable of doing so. Gluten doesn't seem to affect me the way it used to so I am more lax with eating that way. Of course, another reason I stopped eating most gluten free foods is because they are mostly made with rice grain, which is harder on blood sugar. So, I am looking at eating grain free all together. And that, my friend, is hard to do. But I am determined to make this diabetes

My Journey to Better Health

journey without the aid of medicine. So, I will try my best at eating differently; even though this is especially hard to master when everyone else in your house is a carb junkie.

My husband was raised on rice and gravy, and not brown rice mind you. Sticky, delicious, white rice was the main staple of most of their family meals growing up. My childhood was different though. We grew up on potatoes, not rice; northern upbringing versus a southern one. Still, carbs were a large part of our lives and yet we were not unhealthy or overweight as kids. My weight issues all started after my hysterectomy. Again, proof that when we remove the things that God puts in us, we have problems. Now, I had no choice but to have the procedure done, but I will forever struggle with problems because of it, which leads me back to being consistent.

Earlier I spoke to you about nutritional supplements and how they saved me. But I had to be consistent with taking them. I was taking eighty pills a day. Yes, you read that correctly. They were broken up into three times a day, but I did this because I felt so much better with the supplementation. It became common place and not so difficult to take that many pills. It was food-based nutrition and they truly made a huge difference in me. After years of doing this though, it became much harder. You see, I am a gagger. I gag brushing my teeth sometimes. I gag at the dentist office as they clean my teeth. I gag when something does not taste good, and even the thought of some things make me gag. So, swallowing all those pills at times made me gag, and then that reflex got even worse. I truly believe my body was beginning to level out and it just didn't need all of that supplementation anymore. I was always trying to find ways to try to stop taking all those pills anyway. Not that they were doing me harm, quite the opposite. But taking all that was exhausting, especially trying to remember to do it, and affording them was the hardest part of it all.

This is where needing others comes in. You can't learn about new helpful things without researching what others have discovered or by talking to someone who has been through something already. They have the experience to possibly help you in some way, so when others tell their story, someone else benefits from that experience. And I'm not just speaking of physical help here, but mental and spiritual as well.

If I had actually listened better when my sister sent me the information on the adverse effects of diet drinks, then perhaps I wouldn't have gotten to such a low point.

I struggled mentally, physically, and emotionally for the entire length of my children's home-schooling years. Things would irrationally upset me and I had a hard time controlling my emotions and temper. On top of all of this, I knew I was acting irrationally, but was powerless to change my reactions. Being like that made me even more angry and I felt ridiculous about how I reacted, retreating into myself, and hiding away for a while until those feelings would subside. It was a vicious cycle. I avoided many situations because I was uncertain how I would handle or react to them. I avoided conflicts and upsetting others, to the detriment of my own health, all because my emotional state was so raw. I still to this day have a hard time letting people know how I feel about things, but that stems from the way I was

My Journey to Better Health

raised. I was so used to keeping things hidden that I didn't know how to let them go. I still usually handle things privately, within my own mind, whether or not that is proper. But I have come to a point in my life where I do speak out more when someone has upset me or I feel they are wrong. I no longer fear being left or reciprocated upon. I'm not sure if it is age or a better balance of my hormones, or accepting that I can't control other people's choices, only my own. I figure it's a little of all the above. And I figure as long as I stay within God's law and I am grateful for it, people will just have to adjust to this new me..

This does not give me a license to be ugly, but I tend to be very frank at times. Life, I have discovered, is a continual work in progress. Once I get something figured out, it throws me another loop, and I have to reconfigure. But that's okay as long as I continue to make sure I am caring for myself in the process, treating those in my life with the love and respect I myself would want, and trying to make certain that whatever path I am taking; it's the one God has put me on. Because regardless of whatever else I do, I want to please God.

Is my health perfect? Not by far, but I am still, and will likely always be, trying to navigate my crazy, ever-changing body, and let's face it ladies, we have a lot going on in our bodies and all around us, therefore there is a lot that can get off track. And although I may still deal with some issues, I am much farther than I was before. And as long as I continue to try to be a better me, I feel that I am accomplishing something. Don't give up on yourself. Keep fighting for you, your loved ones, your own future. You are worth it. Keep trying to figure out what helps you and what makes you a better person mentally, physically, emotionally, and spiritually. Try to recognize when your day is off and your behavior or actions are not how you would typically react. This is when you learn to change things; when you know something isn't right and you take that next step to correct it.

God did not create us with a spirit of timidity. He made us to prosper and to be bold.

Romans 8:31 says:

> *If God is for us, who can be against us?*

Joshua 1:9 says: Jesus speaking,

> *"I've commanded you, haven't I? Be strong and courageous. Don't be fearful or discouraged because the Lord your God is with you wherever you go."*

Be bold for yourself through Jesus Christ. Glorify Him in all that you undertake. Make better choices. Even if you screw up, tomorrow is another day to begin again. Forgive yourself, take each day one at a time, and renew yourself each morning with the rising of the sun. God has blessed you with one more day. Use it well.

Best regards and many blessings.

About the Author

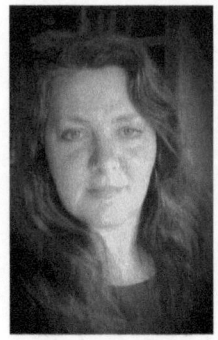

Shawna Boudreaux is a stay at home, home-schooling mom, who started writing books that cover the genres of clean fiction, fantasy, time-travel, and clean-romance novels, within the same book cover, in 2017 after an urging from God. During the process, she has written a total of nine books to date. She has experienced many different health issues, challenges, and trials throughout her life, but with a willingness to try new things, she has also experienced many good things and has been used by God in many different ways over the years. She and her husband of over twenty-five years has lived in the Ragley area north of Lake Charles for their entire married life. They have three children, the youngest a special needs child and forever student. Shawna believes that life is always a learning experience and you should never feel too old to learn something new or follow your dreams.

For other books written by her using her pen name, S.G. Boudreaux, check out her pages on her social media accounts on Facebook, Instagram, Twitter, and her Amazon author page at:
https://www.amazon.com/~/e/B07L525K1X.

You can find more information about her on her website, contact her directly through her Contact the Author page, and also get author signed copies of her fiction works directly from her at https://www.sgboudreaux.com

My Journey to Better Health

www.ingramcontent.com/pod-product-compliance
Lightning Source LLC
Chambersburg PA
CBHW030914080526
44589CB00010B/301